FODMAP
Navigator

Foreword

Gastrointestinal symptoms such as heartburn, bloating, flatulence, abdominal pain, abdominal cramps and diarrhea are uncomfortable and highly prevalent. One reason for this high prevalence is our daily diet.

Western diet is changing and our modern diet is a challenge to the stomach and the intestines. An apple or a glass of orange juice may be healthy, this is not questioned here, but both may promote symptoms of the digestive tract.

Our modern diet contains many ingredients that may cause symptoms attributed to the digestive tract. The term FODMAP stands for fermentable oligo-, di-, and monosaccharides and polyols. In simple words FODMAPs are short-chain carbohydrates and sugar alcohols. These FODMAPs are part of our daily diet, and these FODMAPs were identified to cause gastrointestinal symptoms. The more FODMAPs we consume, the more symptoms we will have.

Reducing daily FODMAP intake will help you to control your gastrointestinal symptoms and may even prevent such symptoms.

In order to maintain a low-FODMAP diet, it is inevitable to know the FODMAP content of all foods. In this FODMAP navigator you will find the ratings for more than 500 foods, food additives and prebiotics.

For questions on missing products please feel free to request information using the email fodmapnavigator@gmail.com.

Martin Storr
fodmapnavigator@gmail.com

MARTIN STORR, MD

FODMAP
Navigator

Low-FODMAP Diet charts with ratings of
more than 500 foods,
food additives and prebiotics

DIGESTA

Table of contents

The FODMAP basics

1) FODMAP stands for fermentable oligo-, di- and monosaccharides and polyols. This means FODMAPs are short-chain carbohydrates and simple sugar alcohols.

2) FODMAPs are normal constituents of our daily diet.

3) FODMAPs may cause abdominal symptoms like increased gas, bloating, flatulence and abdominal pain, soft and frequent stools, diarrhea or constipation, and may worsen pre-existing symptoms.

4) A reduction of the daily amount of consumed FODMAPs helps to reduce these symptoms.

5) In order to consume low-FODMAP foods it is imperative to know the FODMAP content of the foods.

6) Using the FODMAP charts you can rate the FODMAP content of food, food additives and prebiotics and the charts will help you with your grocery shopping.

7) The aim is not to live a FODMAP free life. The aim is to control your symptoms by living a low-FODMAP life.

How to begin a low-FODMAP Diet

Basically, there are 2 ways of conducting a low-FODMAP diet.

> 1) You control your symptoms by permanently consuming low-FODMAP foods.
>
> or
>
> 2) You follow a very strict low-FODMAP diet for 4-6 weeks and then you test your individual tolerance to high-FODMAP foods by reintroducing these foods into your low-FODMAP diet.

It's a requirement for both pathways that you inform yourself on the broad principles of the low-FODMAP diet. This education may be directed by a book or by a personal counseling. Don't forget, sufficient knowledge on the low-FODMAP diet basics is mandatory to make your diet successful.

Variant 1 is the easier variant to follow and can be carried out autonomously after reading a low-FODMAP diet guide book.

Variant 2 is somewhat more difficult at the beginning, but in the long term it allows you to consume a broader range of foods. Variant 2 can be performed after reading a low-FODMAP diet guide book. To increase the chances of this variant to be successful, an individual consultation with a doctor or a dietitian may help.

Be realistic!

A low-FODMAP diet is one way to help you to control your symptoms. But even the best diet may be unable to achieve miracles. Despite being on a low-FODMAP diet there will be the one or the other bad day where your symptoms drive you crazy. Significantly reduced and significantly milder symptoms, that's a realistic goal. If you have realistic expectations towards the low-FODMAP diet, you will be delighted experiencing the achieved improvements and less disappointed by the bad days.

Apart from the FODMAP-content of the consumed food additional individual food intolerances may be present. It is sometimes difficult to identify such personal food intolerances. Some of these individual intolerances may be obvious to you and may be easy to identify. In such cases symptoms occur shortly after consuming the suspected food. If you encounter such individual intolerances, such foods should be avoided.

However, some of these individual intolerances may not be easy to identify. This occurs when foods you may be intolerant to unfold their incompatibilities in the large intestine, likewise to the FODMAPs. Foods usually reach the large intestine many hours after they were consumed and remain in the large intestine, where they cause symptoms, for up to 3 days. Therefore, bloating and other digestive problems may be a consequence to food that you have eaten up to 3 days ago. Now you understand why some food intolerances are not that easy to identify.

Understanding the low-FODMAP diet

For some foods, for example water, FODMAP assessment is easy. Water is low-FODMAP, better said, water is FODMAP-free.

An easy to assess high-FODMAP food is for example high-fructose-corn-syrup (HFCS), which is rated high due to the excessive fructose.

But for numerous foods, the changeover from low-FODMAP to high-FODMAP is fluent. A good example for this fluent transition is the assessment of nuts. While a small amount of nuts is usually well tolerated in a low-FODMAP diet and the amount of FODMAPs consumed is acceptable, a larger amount of nuts is less well tolerated and the amount of FODMAPs has to be rated as being high.

The FODMAP assessment of each food has to be seen in this context. It's best to eat a balanced and varied diet on a low-FODMAP rating. Such a varied low-FODMAP diet will help you to make your diet successful, whereas larger servings of one low-FODMAP food may generate symptoms due to accumulating FODMAPs.

And remain to be honest to yourself. If you were cheating on your diet and consumed an apple, maybe you were craving for this apple, this will not necessarily be a disaster. The symptoms that occur in consequence have to be honestly attributed to the apple and should not be judged as a failure of FODMAP diet. You know exactly why your symptoms returned and you know exactly how to return on the symptom free alley. It was the apple!

The low-FODMAP diet is a new diet, give it a reasonable chance!

The low-FODMAP diet is a very new diet and in addition to scientific food ratings it is to some extent driven by user's experiences, their finest low-FODMAP recipes and user's questions and discussions towards unrated or even possibly wrong rated foods.

These questions and experiences can be read and shared in numerous FODMAP blogs in the www. Just go for this valuable information and contribute to these blogs by posting your own experiences!

For suggestions towards the FODMAP charts, for sharing your finest low-FODMAP recipe or questions on still not rated foods please feel also free to contact the e-mail fodmapnavigator@gmail.com.

The low-FODMAP diet is able to help many but unfortunately not everybody. Reading the clinical trials in which the diet was tested, approximately 80% of the patients with irritable bowel syndrome or related symptoms experienced improvements to their symptoms if they followed the low-FODMAP diet consequently. This means that sensational four out of five had improved symptoms while following a low-FODMAP diet.

Fruits with a high-FODMAP content

Apple
Apricot
Avocado
Blackberry
Boysenberry
Cherry
Currant
Date
Fig
Gooseberry
Guava
Jostaberry
Kaki
Longan fruit
Lychee
Mango
Mirabelle
Nashi pear (Asian pear)
Nectarine
Peach
Pear
Persimmon
Plum
Pomegranate
Prune
Quince
Rambutan
Sharon fruit
Tamarillo
Watermelon

Dried fruit

Vegetables with a high-FODMAP content

Artichoke
Asparagus
Bean (except common bean)
Beetroot
Bell pepper (green)
Brussels sprouts
Cabbage
Cauliflower
Celery root
Chickpea (more than 15 pieces)
Chicoryroot
Corn
Dandelion
Edamame bean
Garlic
Jerusalem artichoke
Leek
Lentil
Mushroom
Onion
Pea
Radicchio
Salsify root
Savoy cabbage
Shallot
Soybean
Spring onion (white part)
Squash, butternut (< 200 g)
Sugar pea

Grains, flours and alternatives with a high-FODMAP content

Barley
Bread (barley/rye/wheat)
Bulgur (wheat)
Cake (grain)
Cereals (grain/dried fruit/honey)
Cookies (grain)
Couscous (wheat)
Fitness bread (grain/fructose/dried fruit)
Gnocchi (wheat)
Gram flour
Kamut (wheat)
Khorasan (wheat)
Lupine flour
Mie noodles (wheat)
Muesli (grain/dried fruit/honey)
Muesli bread (grain/dried fruit/honey)
Noodles/pasta (wheat)
Pastry (grain)
Pie (grain)
Ramen-noodles (wheat)
Rye
Semolina (wheat)
Somen-noodles (wheat)
Soy flour (> 100 gram)
Tortilla (wheat)
Triticale
Udon-noodles (wheat)
Wheat

Dairy foods and dairy alternatives with a high-FODMAP content

Ayran
Blue cheese
Buttermilk
Cheese fondue
Chocolate (milk)
Coffee cream
Coffee whitener
Condensed milk
Cottage cheese
Cow milk
Cream
Cream cheese
Cream yogurt
Creme fraiche
Curd
Ice cream
Kefir
Lassi
Mascarpone
Milk (cow, sheep, goat, donkey)
Milk chocolate
Milk powder
Nougat-cream
Oatmilk
Processed cheese
Pudding
Ricotta cheese
Sheep milk
Soft cheese
Sour cream
Soured milk
Soy milk, from soy beans
Soy cream, from soy beans
Soy yogurt, Yofu
Tzatziki

Whey
Whey cheese
Whey powder
Whipping cream
White chocolate
Yogurt, 1.5% fat
Yogurt, 3.5% fat

Sugars and sweeteners with a high-FODMAP content

Agave syrup
Artificial sweeteners (ending with –ol)
Birch sugar
Corn syrup
Erythritol (E968)
Fructose
Fructose syrup
Glucose-fructose syrup (GFS)
Glycerol (E422)
High-fructose-corn-syrup (HFCS)
Honey
Invert sugar (and additive invertase, E1103)
Isoglucose
Isomaltol (E953)
Lactitol (E966)
Lactose
Maltitol (E965)
Mannitol (E421)
Nougat
Sorbitol (E420)
Thickened pear juice
Xylitol (E967)
Yacon sugar

Other foods with a high-FODMAP content

Applesauce
Barbeque sauce
Broth
Canned fruit
Chutney
Curry sauce
Custard
Fruit concentrate
Fruit juice concentrate
Ketchup
Quorn
Salad dressing (ready-to use)
Sauces (ready-to-eat sauces)
Sauerkraut
Soup powder
Soy burger, veggie burger
Soy chips
Stock cube
Sweet and sour sauce
Tofu, silken
Tomato concentrate

Beverages with a high-FODMAP content

Apple juice
Carob powder Tea (> 1 teaspoons))
Cereal coffee
Chai tea (strong steep)
Chamomile tea
Chicory coffee
Coffee substitute
Energy drink
Fennel tea
Fruit juice (> 125 ml)
Fruit tea (strong steep)
Herbal tea (strong steep)
Lemonade (sweeteners/HFCS)
Malt coffee
Mango juice
Multivitamin juice
Oolong tea
Orange juice
Pear juice

Alcoholic beverages with a high-FODMAP content

Beer (> 1 serving)
Liqueur
Liqueur wine
Port wine
Rum
Sherry
Sparkling wine (semidry, sweet)
Wine (semidry sweet)

Nuts and seeds with a high-FODMAP content

Cashew
Nuts (> 15 pieces)
Pistachio
Seeds (> 15 gram)

Food additives and prebiotics with a high-FODMAP content

Inulin
Lactulose
Polydextrose (E1200)
Raffinose
Stachyose

Spices with a high-FODMAP content

Horseradish
Wasabi

Meat with a high-FODMAP content

Tinned fish (fructose/onion/vegetable powder)
Sausages (lactose/onion/vegetable powder)

Fruits with a low-FODMAP content

Banana
Black raspberry
Blueberry
Canary melon (winter melon)
Cantaloupe
Chestnut
Clementine
Coconut
Cranberry
Dragon fruit (pitaya)
Durian fruit
Galia melon
Grape
Grapefruit
Honeydew
Huckleberry
Jackfruit
Kiwi
Kumquat
Lemon
Lime
Lingonberry
Loganberry
Orange fruit
Oroblanco
Papaya
Passion fruit
Pawpaw
Pineapple
Pomelo
Prickly pear fruit
Raspberry
Rhubarb
Rose hip
Star fruit (carambola)
Strawberry
Tangelo fruit
Tangerine

Vegetables with a low-FODMAP content

Alfalfa
Arugula salad
Aubergine (eggplant)
Bamboo shoot
Beansprouts
Bell pepper (yellow/red)
Bok choy
Broccoli
Carrot
Cassava
Celery stalks
Chard
Cherry tomato
Chickpea (< 15 pieces)
Chicroy leaves
Chillies
Chinese cabbage
Chive
Common bean (string bean, garden bean)
Corn (< 200 gram)
Corn salad (field salad)
Cucumber
Endive
Fennel
Garden cress
Ginger
Iceberg lettuce
Jalapeno pepper
Kohlrabi (turnip cabbage)
Lettuce
Nori algae
Okra
Olive
Parsley
Parsnip
Peperoni
Plantain

Potato
Pumpkin
Radish
Romaine lettuce
Rutabaga (swede)
Seaweed
Soy sprouts
Spinach
Spring onion (green part)
Squash, spaghettisquash, hokkaido
Sweet potato
Taro
Tomato
Turnip
Water chestnut
Watercress
White cabbage
Yams
Zucchini

Grains, flours and alternatives with a low-FODMAP content

Amaranth (pigweed)
Arrowroot
Buckwheat
Chia seeds
Corn flour
Corn starch
Cornmeal
Flax seeds
Millet
Muesli (no wheat, no dried fruit)
Oat
Oat bran
Oatmeal
Polenta
Potato starch
Psyllium (ispaghula)
Quinoa
Rice
Rice flour
Rice starch
Sago
Sorghum
Spelt
Spelt flakes
Starch
Tapioca (manihot)
Teff
Wheat starch

Gluten-free bread
Gluten-free flour
Gluten-free pastry

Buckwheat noodles
Corn noodles
Glass noodles
Gluten-free noodles
Rice noodles
Soba noodles

Cereals (corn/rice/oat)
Corn chips (small serving)
Cornflakes (small serving)
Popcorn
Potato chips (small serving)
Puffed rice
Rice cake
Rice chips
Rice cracker
Taco
Tortilla
Tortilla chips

Watch for high-FODMAP ingredients like sweeteners, fruits and fruit-concentrates in gluten-free products. The soy flour content in gluten-free products, used in a low-FODMAP diet, should not exceed 25%.

The FODMAP content in bakery products is dependent on the fermentation duration of the dough. Short fermentation results in high, long fermentation in low FODMAP content. Ask your baker about fermentation times of his doughs and chose bakery products made from dough with long fermentation time. Bakery produkts from in shop bakeries and industrial sources are economically optimized with short fermentation times and in consequence substantially higher FODMAP content.

Dairy foods and alternatives with a low-FODMAP content

Almond milk
Butter
Buttermilk, lactose free
Coconut milk (< 150 ml)
Coconut water (< 150 ml)
Concentrated butter
Cream, lactose-free
Curd, lactose-free
Hempmilk
Ice cream, lactose-free
Kefir, lactose-free
Margarine
Milk, lactose-free
Milkprotein, casein
Quinoa milk
Rice milk
Sorbet (check fruits)
Soy milk, from soy protein
Wheyprotein
Yogurt, lactose-free

Cheese with a low-FODMAP content

Brie cheese
Butter cheese
Camembert
Cheddar
Chester
Edam
Emmenthal
Feta
Gorgonzola
Gouda
Halloumi
Havarti
Mountain cheese
Mozzarella
Parmesan
Pecorino
Raclette
Ripened cheese
Tilsit

Sugars and sweeteners with a low-FODMAP content

Acesulfame (E905)
Aspartame (E951)
Aspartame-acesulfame (E962)
Brown sugar
Cane sugar (saccharose)
Coconut sugar
Cyclamate (E952)
Dextrose (grape sugar)
Glucose (grape sugar)
Grape sugar (glucose/dextrose)
Icing sugar
Maple syrup
Molasses
Neohesperidine-dihydrochalcone (E959)
Neotame (E961)
Palm sugar
Rice syrup
Saccharin (E954)
Saccharose
Stevia (E960)
Sucralose (E955)
Sucrose
Sugar (sucrose)
Sugar beet syrup
Sugar syrup
Thaumatin (E957)

Meat and animal products with a low-FODMAP content

Bacon
Beef
Chicken
Duck fat
Eggs
Fish
Goose fat
Ham
Lamb
Lard
Pork
Poultry
Seafood
Turkey

Other foods with a low-FODMAP content

Canned tomatoes
Canola oil
Chocolate (dark)
Chocolate drink (watch for milk)
Cocoa
Coconut oil
Cream of coconut
Fish sauce
Garlic oil
Jam (check fruits)
Marmalade
Mayonnaise (< 3 tablespoons)
Miso
Mustard
Olive oil
Oyster sauce
Peanut butter
Salt
Soy oil
Soy protein
Soy sauce
Tahini (< 3 tablespoons)
Tempeh
Tofu, regular, hard
Vegetable oil
Vinegar
Worcestershire sauce
Yeast

Beverages with a low-FODMAP content

Black tea (weak steep)
Bubble tea
Carob powder tea (< 1 teaspoon)
Carrot juice
Chai tea (weak steep)
Coffee (pure coffee)
Cranberry juice
Dandelion tea (weak steep)
Flavored water
Fruit tea (weak steep)
Green tea
Herbal tea (weak steep)
Kombucha
Lemon juice
Lemonades (check for sweeteners)
Liquor (except rum)
Mineral water
Peppermint tea
Rooibos tea
Water
White tea

Alcoholic beverages with a low-FODMAP content

Beer (up to 1 serving)
Gin
Sparkling wine (dry)
Vodka
Whiskey
Wine (dry)

Spices and herbs with a low-FODMAP content

Chili
Herbs, fresh or dried
Lemongrass
Mint
Spices, fresh or dried
Tamarind

Nuts and seeds with a low-FODMAP content

Less than 15 pieces:
Almond
Hazelnut
Walnut

Up to 15 gram:
Brazil nut
Peanut
Pine nut
Poppy seed
Pumpkin seeds
Sesame
Sunflower seed

Food additives with a low-FODMAP content

Acidity regulators (E300-E392, E500-E585)
Agar Agar (E406)
Anti-caking agents (E500-E585)
Anti-foaming agents (E900, E995a)
Antioxidants (E300-E392)
Baking powder
Baking soda (Natron) (E500)
Carboxymethyl cellulose (CMC) (E466)
Carob bean gum (E410)
Carrageen (E407)
Cream stabilizer
Emulsifiers (E322 and E400-E 495)
Ethyl methyl cellulose (E465)
Firming agents (E500-E599)
Flavor enhancers (E620-650)
Foaming agents (E999)
Food colors (E100-E180)
Gases (E938-E949)
Gelatin (E441)
Gelling agents (E400-E495)
Glazing agents, Waxes, Oils (E900-E914)
Guar gum (E412)
Modified starches (E1404-E1451)
Pectin (E440)
Preservatives (E200-E297 and E1105)
Propellants (E941-E946)
Sequestrants (E333, E385, E386, E509, E575-E577)
Sodium carbonate (E500)
Stabilizers (E400-E495)
Thickeners (E400-E495)
Tragacanth (E413)
Xanthan gum (E415)

Alphabetic list of foods, food additives and prebiotics with high or low-FODMAP rating

Acesulfame (E905)	low
Acidity regulators (E300-E392, E500-E585)	low
Agar Agar (E406)	low
Agave syrup	high
Alfalfa	low
Almond (< 15 pieces)	low
Almond milk	low
Amaranth (pigweed)	low
Anti-caking agents (E500-E585)	low
Anti-foaming agents (E900, E995a)	low
Antioxidants (E300-E392)	low
Apple	high
Apple juice	high
Applesauce	high
Apricot	high
Arrowroot	low
Artichoke	high
Artificial sweeteners (ending with –ol)	high
Arugula salad	low
Asparagus	high
Aspartame (E951)	low
Aspartame-acesulfame (E962)	low
Aubergine (eggplant)	low
Avocado	high
Ayran	high
Bacon	low
Baking powder	low
Baking soda (Natron)(E500)	low
Bamboo shoot	low
Banana	low

Barbeque sauce	high
Barley	high
Birch sugar	high
Bean (except common bean)	high
Beansprouts	low
Beef	low
Beer (> 1 serving)	high
Beer (up to 1 serving)	low
Beetroot	high
Bell pepper (green)	high
Bell pepper (yellow/red)	low
Black raspberry	low
Black tea (weak steep)	low
Blackberry	high
Blue cheese	high
Blueberry	low
Bok choy	low
Boysenberry	high
Brasil nut (< 15 g)	low
Bread (barley/rye/wheat)	high
Brie cheese	low
Broccoli	low
Broth	high
Brown sugar	low
Brussels sprouts	high
Bubble tea	low
Buckwheat	low
Buckwheat noodles	low
Bulgur (wheat)	high
Butter	low
Butter cheese	low
Buttermilk	high
Cabbage	high
Cake (grain)	high

Camembert	low
Canary melon (winter melon)	low
Cane sugar (saccharose)	low
Canned fruit	high
Canned tomatoes	low
Canola oil	low
Cantaloupe	low
Carboxymethyl cellulose (CMC)(E466)	low
Carob bean gum (E410)	low
Carob powder tea (< 1 teaspoon)	low
Carob powder tea (> 2 teaspoons)	high
Carrageen (E407)	low
Carrot	low
Carrot juice	low
Cashew	high
Cassava	low
Cauliflower	high
Celery root	high
Celery stalks	low
Cereal coffee	high
Cereals (corn/rice/oat)	low
Cereals (grain/dried fruit/honey)	high
Chai tea (strong steep)	high
Chai tea (weak steep)	low
Chamomile tea	high
Chard	low
Cheddar	low
Cheese fondue	high
Cherry	high
Cherry tomato	low
Chester	low
Chestnut	low
Chia seeds	low
Chicken	low

Chickpea (< 15 pieces)	low
Chickpea (more than 15 pieces)	high
Chicoryroot	high
Chicory leaves	low
Chicory coffee	high
Chili	low
Chinese cabbage	low
Chive	low
Chocolate (dark)	low
Chocolate (milk)	high
Chocolate drink (watch for milk)	low
Chutney	high
Clementine	low
Cocoa	low
Coconut	low
Coconut milk	low
Coconut oil	low
Coconut sugar	low
Coconut water	low
Coffee (pure coffee)	low
Coffee cream	high
Coffee substitute	high
Coffee whitener	high
Common bean (string bean, garden bean)	low
Concentrated butter	low
Condensed milk	high
Cookies (grain)	high
Corn	high
Corn (< 200 gram)	low
Corn chips (small serving)	low
Corn flour	low
Corn salad (field salad)	low
Corn starch	low
Corn syrup	high

Cornflakes (small serving)	low
Cornmeal	low
Cottage cheese	high
Couscous (wheat)	high
Cow milk	high
Cranberry	low
Cranberry juice	low
Cream	high
Cream cheese	high
Cream of coconut	low
Cream stabilizer	low
Cream yogurt	high
Cream, lactose-free	low
Creme fraiche	high
Cucumber	low
Curd	high
Curd, lactose-free	low
Currant	high
Curry sauce	high
Custard	high
Cyclamate (E952)	low
Dandelion	high
Dandelion tea (weak steep)	low
Date	high
Dextrose (grape sugar)	low
Dragon fruit (Pitaya)	low
Dried fruit	high
Duck fat	low
Durian fruit	low
Edam	low
Edamame bean	high
Eggs	low
Emmenthal	low
Emulsifiers (E322 and E400-E 495)	low

Endive	low
Energy drink	high
Erythritol (E968)	high
Ethyl methyl cellulose (E465)	low
Fennel	low
Fennel tea	high
Feta	low
Fig	high
Firming agents (E500-E599)	low
Fish	low
Fish sauce	low
Fitness bread (grain/fructose/dried fruit)	high
Flavor enhancers (E620-650)	low
Flavored water	low
Flax seeds	low
Foaming agents (E999)	low
Food colors (E100-E180)	low
Fructose	high
Fructose syrup	high
Fruit concentrate	high
Fruit juice (> 125 ml)	high
Fruit juice concentrate	high
Fruit tea (strong steep)	high
Fruit tea (weak steep)	low
Galia melon	low
Garden cress	low
Garlic	high
Garlic oil	low
Gases (E938-E949)	low
Gelatin (E441)	low
Gelling agents (E400-E495)	low
Gin	low
Ginger	low
Glass noodles	low

Glazing agents, waxes, oils (E900-E914)	low
Glucose (grape sugar)	low
Glucose-fructose syrup (GFS)	high
Gluten-free bread	low
Gluten-free flour	low
Gluten-free noodles	low
Gluten-free pastry	low
Glycerol (E422)	high
Gnocchi (wheat)	high
Goose fat	low
Gooseberry	high
Gorgonzola	low
Gouda	low
Gram flour	high
Grape	low
Grape sugar (glucose/dextrose)	low
Grapefruit	low
Green tea	low
Guar gum (E412)	low
Guava	high
Halloumi	low
Ham	low
Havarti	low
Hazelnut (< 15 pieces)	low
Hemp milk	low
Herbal tea (strong steep)	high
Herbal tea (weak steep)	low
Herbs, fresh or dried	low
High-fructose-corn-syrup (HFCS)	high
Honey	high
Honeydew	low
Horseradish	high
Huckleberry	low
Ice cream	high

Ice cream, lactose-free	low
Iceberg lettuce	low
Icing sugar	low
Inulin	high
Invert sugar (and additive invertase, E1103)	high
Isoglucose	high
Isomaltol (E953)	high
Jackfruit	low
Jalapeno pepper	low
Jam (check fruits)	low
Jerusalem artichoke	high
Jostaberry	high
Kaki	high
Kamut (wheat)	high
Kefir	high
Kefir, lactose-free	low
Ketchup	high
Khorasan (wheat)	high
Kiwi	low
Kohlrabi (turnip cabbage)	low
Kombucha	low
Kumquat	low
Lactitol (E966)	high
Lactose	high
Lactulose	high
Lamb	low
Lard	low
Lassi	high
Leek	high
Lemon	low
Lemon juice	low
Lemonade (sweeteners/HFCS)	high
Lemonades (check for sweeteners)	low
Lemongrass	low

Lentil	high
Lettuce	low
Lime	low
Lingonberry	low
Liqueur	high
Liqueur wine	high
Liquor (except rum)	low
Loganberry	low
Longan fruit	high
Lupine flour	high
Lychee	high
Malt coffee	high
Maltitol (E965)	high
Mango	high
Mango juice	high
Mannitol (E421)	high
Maple syrup	low
Margarine	low
Marmalade	low
Mascarpone	high
Mayonnaise (< 3 tablespoons)	low
Mie noodles (wheat)	high
Milk (cow, sheep, goat, donkey)	high
Milk chocolate	high
Milk powder	high
Milk protein	low
Milk, lactose-free	low
Millet	low
Mineral water	low
Mint	low
Mirabelle	high
Miso	low
Modified starches (E1404-E1451)	low
Molasses	low

Mountain cheese	low
Mozzarella	low
Muesli (grain/dried fruit/honey)	high
Muesli (no wheat, no dried fruit)	low
Muesli bread (grain/dried fruit/honey)	high
Multivitamin juice	high
Mushroom	high
Mustard	low
Nashi pear (Asian pear)	high
Nectarine	high
Neohesperidine-dihydrochalcone (E959)	low
Neotame (E961)	low
Noodles/pasta (wheat)	high
Nori algae	low
Nougat	high
Nougat-cream	high
Nuts (> 15 pieces)	high
Oat	low
Oat bran	low
Oat milk	high
Oatmeal	low
Okra	low
Olive	low
Olive oil	low
Onion	high
Oolong tea	high
Orange fruit	low
Orange juice	high
Oroblanco	low
Oyster sauce	low
Palm sugar	low
Papaya	low
Parmesan	low
Parsley	low

Parsnip	low
Passion fruit	low
Pastry (grain)	high
Pawpaw	low
Pea	high
Peach	high
Peanut (up to 15 gram)	low
Peanut butter	low
Pear	high
Pear juice	high
Pecorino	low
Pectin (E440)	low
Peperoni	low
Peppermint tea	low
Persimmon	high
Pie (grain)	high
Pine nut (up to 15 gram)	low
Pineapple	low
Pistachio	high
Plantain	low
Plum	high
Polenta	low
Polydextrose (E1200)	high
Pomegranate	high
Pomelo	low
Popcorn	low
Poppy seed (< 15 g)	low
Pork	low
Port wine	high
Potato	low
Potato chips (small serving)	low
Potato starch	low
Poultry	low
Preservatives (E200-E297 and E1105)	low

Prickly pear fruit	low
Processed cheese	high
Propellants (E941-E946)	low
Prune	high
Psyllium (ispaghula)	low
Pudding	high
Puffed rice	low
Pumpkin	low
Pumpkin seeds (up to 15 gram)	low
Quince	high
Quinoa	low
Quinoa milk	low
Quorn	high
Raclette	low
Radicchio	high
Radish	low
Raffinose	high
Rambutan	high
Ramen-noodles (wheat)	high
Raspberry	low
Rhubarb	low
Rice	low
Rice cake	low
Rice chips	low
Rice cracker	low
Rice flour	low
Rice milk	low
Rice noodles	low
Rice starch	low
Rice syrup	low
Ricotta cheese	high
Ripened cheese	low
Rooibos tea	low
Romaine lettuce	low

Rose hip	low
Rum	high
Rutabaga (swede)	low
Rye	high
Saccharin (E954)	low
Saccharose	low
Sago	low
Salad dressing (ready-to use)	high
Salsify root	high
Salt	low
Sauces (ready-to-eat sauces)	high
Sauerkraut	high
Sausages (lactose/onion/vegetable powder)	high
Savoy cabbage	high
Seafood	low
Seaweed	low
Seeds (> 15 gram)	high
Semolina (wheat)	high
Sequestrants (E333, E385, E386, E509, E575-	low
Sesame (up to 15 gram)	low
Shallot	high
Sharon fruit	high
Sheep milk	high
Sherry	high
Soba noodles	low
Sodium carbonate (E500)	low
Soft cheese	high
Somen-noodles (wheat)	high
Sorbet (check fruits)	low
Sorbitol (E420)	high
Sorghum	low
Soup powder	high
Sour cream	high
Soured milk	high

Soy burger, veggie burger	high
Soy chips	high
Soy flour (> 100 gram)	high
Soy cream, from soy beans	high
Soy milk, from soy protein	low
Soy milk, from soy beans	high
Soy oil	low
Soy protein	low
Soy yogurt	high
Soy sauce	low
Soybean	high
Sparkling wine (dry)	low
Sparkling wine (semidry, sweet)	high
Spelt	low
Spelt flakes	low
Spices, fresh or dried	low
Spinach	low
Spring onion (green part)	low
Spring onion (white part)	high
Squash, butternut (< 200 g)	low
Squash, butternut (< 200 g)	low
Squash, lokkaido, spaghettisquash	low
Stabilizers (E400-E495)	low
Stachyose	high
Star fruit (carambola)	low
Starch	low
Stevia (E960)	low
Stock cube	high
Strawberry	low
Sucralose (E955)	low
Sucrose	low
Sugar (sucrose)	low
Sugar beet syrup	low
Sugar pea	high

Sugar syrup	low
Sunflower seed (up to 15 gram)	low
Sweet and sour sauce	high
Sweet potato	low
Taco	low
Tahini (< 3 tablespoons)	low
Tamarillo	high
Tamarind	low
Tangelo fruit	low
Tangerine	low
Tapioca (manihot)	low
Taro	low
Teff	low
Tempeh	low
Thaumatin (E957)	low
Thickened pear juice	high
Thickeners (E400-E495)	low
Tilsit	low
Tinned fish (fructose/onion/vegetable powder)	high
Tofu, regular, hard	low
Tofu, silken	high
Tomato	low
Tomato concentrate	high
Tortilla	low
Tortilla (wheat)	high
Tortilla chips	low
Tragacanth (E413)	low
Triticale	high
Turkey	low
Turnip	low
Tzatziki	high
Udon-noodles (wheat)	high
Vegetable oil	low
Vinegar	low

Vodka	low
Walnut (< 15 pieces)	low
Wasabi	high
Water	low
Water chestnut	low
Watercress	low
Watermelon	high
Wheat	high
Wheat starch	low
Whey	high
Whey cheese	high
Whey powder	high
Whey protein	low
Whipping cream	high
Whiskey	low
White cabbage	low
White chocolate	high
White tea	low
Wine (dry)	low
Wine (semidry sweet)	high
Worcestershire sauce	low
Xanthan gum (E415)	low
Xylitol (E967)	high
Yacon sugar	high
Yams	low
Yeast	low
Yogurt, 1.5% fat	high
Yogurt, 3.5% fat	high
Yogurt, lactose-free	low
Zucchini	low

Food additives and their European E-xxx numbers that received a FODMAP rating in the FODMAP Navigator

E100-E180	Food colors
E200-E297	Preservatives
E300-E392	Antioxidants, acidity regulators
E400-E495	Thickeners, stabilizers, emulsifiers
E406	Agar Agar
E407	Carrageen
E410	Carob bean gum
E412	Guar gum
E413	Tragacanth
E415	Xanthan gum
E420	Sorbitol
E421	Mannitol
E422	Glycerol
E440	Pectin
E441	Gelatin
E466	Carboxymethyl cellulose (CMC)
E465	Ethyl methyl cellulose
E500	Sodium carbonate
E500-E585	Acidity regulators, anti-caking agents
E620-E650	Flavor enhancers
E900-E914	Glazing agents
E938-E949	Gases
E950-E969	Sweeteners
E950	Acesulfame
E951	Aspartame
E952	Cyclamate
E953	Isomaltol
E954	Saccharin
E955	Sucralose
E957	Thaumatin
E959	Neohesperidine-dihydrochalcone
E960	Stevia
E961	Neotame

E962	Aspartame-acesulfame
E965	Maltitol
E966	Lactitol
E967	Xylitol
E968	Erythritol
E1103	Invertase
E1200	Polydextrose
E1404-E1451	Modified starches

The food additives in the FODMAP-Navigator were evaluated on the background of their suitability within the low-FODMAP diet. Please note that many of these food additives are seen critically in terms of tolerance and hazardousness. Ideally you avoid industrially produced food products which will limit your intake of such food additives.

Books

The charts within the FODMAP-Navigator are meant to be used as a supplement to existing low-FODMAP diet guides or as an addition to your consultation with a physician or dietician. Without guidance the low-FODMAP diet may not be as successful as it could be.

You will find good guidance in the below listed books:

Shepherd, S., Gibson, P., Chey, W.; The Complete Low-FODMAP Diet: A Revolutionary Plan for Managing IBS and Other Digestive Disorders; The Experiment Press (August 2013)

Catsos, P.; IBS: Free at Last! Change Your Carbs, Change Your Life with the FODMAP Elimination Diet; Pond Cove Press (April 2012)

Shepherd, S.; The Low-FODMAP Diet Cookbook: 150 Simple, Flavorful, Gut-Friendly Recipes to Ease the Symptoms of IBS, Celiac Disease, Crohn's Disease, Ulcerative Colitis, and Other Digestive Disorders; The Experiment Press (July 2014)

Bolen, B. and Bradlex, K.; The Everything Guide To The Low-Fodmap Diet: A Healthy Plan for Managing IBS and Other Digestive Disorders; Adams Media (November 2014)

Catsos, P.; Flavor without FODMAPs Cookbook: Love the Foods that Love You Back; Pond Cove Press (February 2014)

Anderson, M.; All about Low-FODMAP Diet & IBS: A Very Quick Guide; Temescal Press (November 2014)

Morgan, D.; The Low FODMAP diet: The Essential Guide and Cookbook to the Most Effective IBS Diet; CreateSpace (January 2015)

FODMAP Apps

There are several Apps on the low-FODMAP diet for Apple and Android available. These Apps include lists of foods with low-FODMAP and high-FODMAP ratings. Some of these Apps give additional information on moderate-FODMAP rating.

Most of these Apps provide information on a limited number of foods. The numbers of rated foods usually ranges from 50-100. Therefore these Apps are suitable for quick but limited information at the grocery store. With these limitations these Apps are currently of limited usefulness.

Most Apps contain food lists only. Some Apps contain to a limited extend some general information on the low-FODMAP diet or some recipes.

Presently the most up to date App seems to be the Monash University low-FODMAP Diet App that can be found here:

http://www.med.monash.edu.au/cecs/gastro/fodmap/iphone-app.html.

57436077R00031

Made in the USA
Middletown, DE
16 December 2017